Carb Cycling Guide for Beginners

Choosing the Right Carb Cycling Plan

By

Bryden Cael

Table of Contents

CHAPTER 1

Introduction

1.1 What is Carb Cycling?

Carb cycling is a dietary strategy that involves varying your daily carbohydrate intake. It's a structured approach where you alternate between days of higher carbohydrate consumption and days of lower carbohydrate consumption. The goal is to optimize the timing and quantity of carbohydrates to meet specific fitness, health, or performance objectives.

In carb cycling, high-carb days are typically referred to as "refeed" days, while low-carb days are often termed "cutting" or "restrictive" days. The distribution of these days can vary depending on individual goals and preferences. Some people may follow a weekly cycle, while others may implement a longer-term pattern, such as a 10-day or 14-day cycle.

During high-carb days, you consume more carbohydrates, which can provide your body with energy and help replenish glycogen stores in your muscles and liver. This can be particularly beneficial for athletes, bodybuilders, and active individuals looking to maximize performance during workouts.

On low-carb days, you reduce your carbohydrate intake, forcing your body to rely on fat for energy instead. This is often used in conjunction with a caloric deficit to promote fat loss. By strategically reducing carbs on these days, you can achieve a calorie deficit, which is fundamental for weight loss.

1.2 Who Should Consider Carb Cycling?

Carb cycling can be an effective dietary approach for various individuals, but it's particularly suited for those with specific goals and needs. Here are some groups who might consider carb cycling:

1. **Athletes and Fitness Enthusiasts**: Carb cycling can be a valuable tool for athletes and individuals engaged in high-intensity workouts. It helps optimize energy levels during training and supports muscle recovery.

2. **Bodybuilders**: Carb cycling is commonly used by bodybuilders, especially during the cutting phase of their training. It allows them to reduce body fat while preserving muscle mass.

3. **Weight Loss Seekers**: Those
    looking to lose weight can
    benefit from carb cycling, as it
    helps control calorie intake,
    manage hunger, and promote fat
    loss when combined with a
    caloric deficit.

4. **Metabolic Adaptation**: People
    who have experienced metabolic
    adaptation (a slowdown in
    metabolism) due to prolonged
    calorie restriction may use carb
    cycling to "reset" their
    metabolism and prevent weight
    loss plateaus.

5. **Endurance Athletes**: Endurance
    athletes like marathon runners
    and triathletes may use carb
    cycling to optimize their
    carbohydrate intake before races
    or long training sessions.

6. **Health-Conscious Individuals**: Even those not primarily focused on performance or weight management can use carb cycling to balance their diet, reduce the risk of insulin resistance, and promote overall health.

7. **People with Specific Dietary Preferences**: Carb cycling can be adapted to various dietary preferences, including vegan, vegetarian, paleo, or gluten-free diets, making it a flexible approach.

1.3 Benefits of Carb Cycling

Carb cycling offers several potential benefits:

1. **Fat Loss**: By strategically reducing carb intake on certain

days, carb cycling can help promote fat loss. Low-carb days create a calorie deficit, leading to a reduction in body fat.

2. **Muscle Preservation**: High-carb days provide the energy needed to support workouts and prevent muscle loss during calorie deficits.

3. **Performance Optimization**: Athletes and active individuals can benefit from increased energy on high-carb days, enhancing their performance during training sessions and competitions.

4. **Metabolic Flexibility**: Carb cycling encourages metabolic flexibility, allowing the body to efficiently use both carbohydrates and fats for energy.

5. **Blood Sugar Control**: For those at risk of or dealing with insulin resistance, carb cycling can help manage blood sugar levels and reduce the risk of related health issues.

6. **Sustainability**: Carb cycling can be more sustainable than long-term low-carb diets for some people, as it provides periodic relief from strict carbohydrate restrictions.

7. **Psychological Benefits**: Knowing that you have both high and low-carb days can make dieting more manageable and less monotonous.

carb cycling is a dietary strategy that involves alternating between high and low-carb days, making it a versatile approach suitable for various individuals, including athletes, weight loss seekers, and health-conscious individuals. The benefits of carb cycling include fat loss, muscle preservation, performance optimization, metabolic flexibility, blood sugar control, sustainability, and psychological advantages, making it a valuable tool in achieving specific health and fitness goals.

CHAPTER 2

Understanding Carbohydrates

2.1 Types of Carbohydrates

Carbohydrates are one of the three main macronutrients, alongside fats and proteins. They are essential for providing energy to the body. Carbohydrates come in various forms, and understanding their types is crucial for making informed dietary choices. Here are the main types of carbohydrates:

- **Simple Carbohydrates**: These are composed of one or two sugar molecules and are quickly digested. Common sources include table sugar (sucrose), fruit sugar (fructose), and milk sugar (lactose).

- **Complex Carbohydrates**: These are made up of long chains of sugar molecules and take longer to break down. They provide sustained energy. Examples include starches found in foods like grains, legumes, and vegetables.

- **Dietary Fiber**: Fiber is a type of complex carbohydrate that the body cannot digest. It's essential for digestive health and is found in foods like whole grains, fruits, vegetables, and legumes.

- **Glycogen**: This is the storage form of carbohydrates in the body, primarily stored in the liver and muscles. It can be quickly converted into glucose to provide energy when needed.

- **Monosaccharides**: These are the
  simplest form of carbohydrates,
  consisting of a single sugar
  molecule. Common
  monosaccharides include
  glucose, fructose, and galactose.

- **Disaccharides**: These are
  composed of two sugar
  molecules. Examples include
  sucrose (glucose + fructose),
  lactose (glucose + galactose),
  and maltose (glucose + glucose).

- **Polysaccharides**: These are long
  chains of sugar molecules,
  making them complex
  carbohydrates. Examples include
  starch, which is the storage form
  of energy in plants, and
  glycogen, the storage form of
  energy in animals.

The different types of carbohydrates is
essential for managing your diet and

making choices that align with your health and fitness goals.

2.2 The Role of Carbohydrates in the Body

Carbohydrates serve several vital roles in the human body:

- **Energy Source**: Carbohydrates are the body's primary source of energy. When consumed, they are broken down into glucose, which is used for immediate energy or stored as glycogen for later use.

- **Brain Fuel**: Glucose derived from carbohydrates is the preferred fuel for the brain. It provides the energy necessary for cognitive functions, concentration, and overall mental well-being.

- **Muscle Function**: Muscles rely on carbohydrates for energy during physical activities. Carbohydrate availability is critical for athletic performance and endurance.

- **Glycogen Storage**: Excess glucose is converted into glycogen and stored in the liver and muscles. This glycogen reserve is crucial for maintaining blood glucose levels and sustaining energy during fasting or physical exertion.

- **Digestive Health**: Dietary fiber, a type of carbohydrate, is essential for digestive health. It promotes regular bowel movements, helps prevent constipation, and supports the growth of beneficial gut bacteria.

- **Blood Sugar Regulation**: Carbohydrates play a role in regulating blood sugar levels. The body's ability to manage glucose effectively is critical for preventing conditions like diabetes.

2.3 Glycemic Index and Carb Selection

The Glycemic Index (GI) is a scale that measures how quickly and significantly a carbohydrate-containing food raises blood sugar levels. Understanding the GI of foods is essential for making informed carbohydrate choices, especially for individuals concerned about blood sugar control or those seeking to optimize their energy intake. Here's a breakdown of the Glycemic Index and carb selection:

- **Low GI Foods**: These are
  carbohydrates that are digested
  and absorbed slowly, resulting in
  a gradual increase in blood sugar
  levels. Foods with a low GI
  include whole grains, legumes,
  non-starchy vegetables, and most
  fruits. Choosing low GI foods
  can help maintain steady energy
  levels and prevent blood sugar
  spikes.

- **Moderate GI Foods**: These
  carbohydrates fall in the middle
  of the GI scale. They include
  foods like whole wheat products
  and some fruits. They have a
  moderate impact on blood sugar
  and can be part of a balanced
  diet.

- **High GI Foods**: High GI
  carbohydrates are rapidly
  digested and cause a quick
  increase in blood sugar levels.

Examples include white bread, sugary cereals, and processed snacks. These foods should be consumed in moderation, especially for those with diabetes or those seeking stable energy levels.

The types of carbohydrates, their roles in the body, and the Glycemic Index can help individuals make informed choices about the carbohydrates they consume. Selecting the right types of carbohydrates can support overall health, energy management, and blood sugar regulation.

CHAPTER 3
The Science of Carb Cycling

3.1 How Carb Cycling Affects Your Body

Carb cycling is a dietary strategy that can have a significant impact on your body's metabolism, energy utilization, and overall health. Here's how carb cycling affects your body:

- **Energy Source Variation**: On high-carb days, your body primarily relies on carbohydrates for energy. This means your glycogen stores are replenished, providing ample energy for intense workouts and daily activities. On low-carb days, when carbohydrates are restricted, your body shifts to using stored fat as its primary energy source. This promotes fat loss and helps maintain muscle mass when combined with a caloric deficit.

- **Metabolic Flexibility**: Carb cycling promotes metabolic flexibility, enabling your body to efficiently use both carbohydrates and fats for energy. This flexibility is advantageous because it allows you to adapt to changing energy demands, whether it's a high-intensity workout or a low-activity rest day.

- **Insulin Sensitivity**: Carb cycling can improve insulin sensitivity, making your body's response to carbohydrates more efficient. This can help regulate blood sugar levels and reduce the risk of insulin resistance, which is associated with type 2 diabetes and other health issues.

- **Hunger and Satiety**: Carb cycling may help manage hunger and satiety. High-carb days can provide a psychological and physiological break from dieting, reducing feelings of deprivation. On low-carb days, the increase in protein and fat intake can promote feelings of fullness and satisfaction.

- **Muscle Preservation**: On high-carb days, you provide your muscles with the glycogen they need for optimal performance and recovery. This can help preserve muscle mass, especially when you're in a calorie deficit during weight loss phases.

- **Calorie Cycling**: Carb cycling inherently involves calorie cycling, as high-carb days typically have more calories than low-carb days. This can prevent your metabolism from adapting to a fixed calorie intake, potentially avoiding the plateau often seen with continuous calorie restriction.

3.2 Metabolic Adaptation

Metabolic adaptation, often referred to as the "starvation mode" or the body's adaptive response to calorie restriction, is a crucial aspect to consider when implementing carb cycling. Here's how carb cycling interacts with metabolic adaptation:

- **Preventing Metabolic Adaptation**: Carb cycling, through its calorie and carbohydrate variations, can help prevent metabolic adaptation to a consistently low-calorie intake. When you restrict calories for extended periods, your metabolism may slow down to conserve energy, making it harder to continue losing weight. Carb cycling disrupts this pattern, potentially helping you maintain a higher metabolic rate.

- **Caloric Surpluses and Deficits**: During high-carb days, you consume more calories, potentially preventing your body from entering a prolonged caloric deficit. This can be particularly advantageous in avoiding metabolic slowdown. On low-carb days, the calorie deficit promotes fat loss without the risk of metabolic adaptation that might occur with a constant low-calorie intake.

- **Adaptation Prevention**: The variation in carbohydrate intake on carb cycling helps avoid metabolic adaptation, keeping your metabolism flexible and responsive to different calorie levels. This adaptability can make weight management more sustainable and effective.

3.3 Hormonal Changes

Carb cycling can influence several hormones in the body, impacting factors such as energy utilization, appetite, and muscle growth. Here are some hormonal changes associated with carb cycling:

- **Insulin**: Insulin is a hormone responsible for regulating blood

sugar levels and nutrient storage.
On high-carb days, insulin levels
tend to increase due to increased
carbohydrate intake. This
promotes the storage of glucose
as glycogen in muscles and the
liver. On low-carb days, insulin
levels decrease, favoring fat
utilization for energy.

- **Leptin**: Leptin is a hormone that
  plays a key role in appetite
  regulation and energy
  expenditure. Carb cycling may
  help prevent leptin levels from
  dropping significantly during
  prolonged calorie deficits.
  Maintaining higher leptin levels
  can help control hunger and
  maintain metabolic rate.

- **Ghrelin**: Ghrelin is a hormone
  that stimulates appetite. Carb
  cycling can influence ghrelin
  levels, potentially reducing

hunger and food cravings on low-carb days, thanks to the satiety-promoting effects of protein and fat.

- **Cortisol**: Cortisol, often referred to as the stress hormone, can be influenced by prolonged calorie deficits. Carb cycling can mitigate the stress response associated with constant low-calorie diets, potentially reducing the release of cortisol and its potential negative effects on muscle preservation.

carb cycling affects the body by altering energy sources, promoting metabolic flexibility, improving insulin sensitivity, managing hunger, and preserving muscle mass. It also plays a role in preventing metabolic adaptation by varying calorie intake and influencing several hormones, which can help maintain a higher metabolic

rate and make weight management
more sustainable.

CHAPTER 4

Getting Started with Carb Cycling

4.1 Setting Your Goals

Getting started with carb cycling begins with setting clear and achievable goals. Your goals will determine the specific approach you take and the structure of your carb cycling plan. Here are some steps to help you set your goals:

- **Define Your Objectives**: Determine what you want to achieve with carb cycling. Are you aiming for fat loss, muscle gain, improved athletic performance, or better blood sugar control? Your goals will guide your carb cycling plan.

- **Establish a Realistic Timeline**: Consider how quickly you want to achieve your goals. Be realistic about the time it will take to see significant changes.

- **Quantify Your Goals**: Make your goals specific and measurable. For example, if your goal is weight loss, specify how many pounds or inches you want to lose.

- **Consider Your Current Lifestyle**: Assess your current diet, exercise routine, and lifestyle. Understand how carb cycling can fit into your daily life.

- **Consult a Healthcare Professional**: If you have specific health concerns or medical conditions, it's advisable to consult a healthcare professional or registered dietitian to ensure your carb cycling plan is safe and suitable for you.

4.2 Choosing the Right Carb Cycling Plan

Once you've set your goals, the next step is to choose the right carb cycling plan that aligns with your objectives. There are various approaches to carb cycling, and the one you select should be tailored to your specific needs. Here are some common carb cycling plans:

- **Classic Carb Cycling**: This plan alternates between high-carb days, low-carb days, and sometimes very low-carb days. It is often used for fat loss and muscle preservation.

- **Bodybuilder Carb Cycling**: Bodybuilders may use a more structured approach, varying their carbohydrate intake based on training days (higher carbs) and rest days (lower carbs). The goal is to support muscle growth and minimize fat gain.

- **Weekly Carb Cycling**: This plan typically involves cycling carbohydrates on a weekly basis. You might have a few days of high-carb intake followed by a few days of low-carb intake in a recurring pattern.

- **Targeted Ketogenic Diet (TKD)**: In TKD, you consume high-carb meals or snacks around your workouts to provide energy for intense training while maintaining a low-carb diet at other times.

- **Cyclical Ketogenic Diet (CKD)**: CKD involves alternating between periods of strict ketogenic (very low-carb) dieting and periods of higher-carb intake. It's often used by individuals following a ketogenic diet but looking to enhance athletic performance.

Choose the plan that aligns with your goals, preferences, and lifestyle. Keep in mind that consistency is crucial, so select a plan that you can sustain over time.

4.3 Meal Planning and Preparation

Effective meal planning and preparation are essential for

successfully implementing a carb cycling plan. Here's how to get started:

- **Calculate Your Macronutrients**: Determine the macronutrient ratios (carbohydrates, proteins, and fats) for each phase of your carb cycling plan. There are various online tools and calculators that can help with this. Make sure your plan supports your goals and provides sufficient nutrients.

- **Create a Meal Schedule**: Plan your high-carb and low-carb days in advance, along with specific meals and snacks. Having a schedule will help you stay on track and prevent impulsive, less healthy choices.

- **Prepare Balanced Meals**: Ensure that each meal contains a balance of protein, carbohydrates, and healthy fats. Include a variety of whole foods such as lean meats, fish, vegetables, fruits, nuts, and whole grains.

- **Stock Up on Food**: Keep your kitchen stocked with the necessary ingredients to make meal preparation convenient. Having healthy foods readily available will make it easier to stick to your plan.

- **Meal Prepping**: Consider preparing meals in advance, especially if you have a busy lifestyle. Cook several meals at once, portion them, and store them in the fridge or freezer. This can help you avoid resorting to less healthy options when you're pressed for time.

- **Track Your Progress**: Keep a food diary or use a mobile app to track your food intake. Monitoring what you eat can help you stay consistent and make adjustments to your plan as needed.

- **Stay Hydrated**: Don't forget about the importance of hydration. Drinking enough water is crucial for overall health and can also help manage hunger and cravings.

By setting clear goals, choosing the right carb cycling plan, and mastering meal planning and preparation, you'll be well on your way to implementing carb cycling successfully and working toward your desired outcomes.

CHAPTER 5

Implementing Your Carb Cycling Plan

5.1 High Carb Days

High carb days are a fundamental component of a carb cycling plan, designed to provide your body with a surplus of carbohydrates to support energy, muscle recovery, and performance. Here's how to implement high carb days effectively:

1. Determine the Frequency:

- Decide how often you'll have high carb days in your carb cycling plan. The frequency can vary based on your goals, but it's typically around 1-3 times per week, depending on your activity level and objectives.

2. Choose Quality Carbohydrate Sources:

- Focus on complex carbohydrates from sources like whole grains (oats, quinoa, brown rice), starchy vegetables (sweet potatoes, squash), legumes (beans, lentils), and fruits. These provide sustained energy and essential nutrients.

3. Time Your High Carb Days:

- Schedule high carb days on days when you have intense workouts, as your body will benefit from the extra energy. They can be especially useful before resistance training sessions or high-intensity interval training (HIIT).

4. Monitor Portions:

- While high carb days involve consuming more carbohydrates, it's still essential to monitor portion sizes. Overeating can lead to an excessive calorie intake, potentially hindering your goals.

5. Include Adequate Protein:

- Don't neglect protein intake on high carb days. Protein is essential for muscle repair and growth. Aim for a balanced meal that includes lean protein sources like chicken, fish, tofu, or legumes.

6. Stay Hydrated:

- Maintain proper hydration, as your body requires water for carbohydrate metabolism. Drink enough water throughout the day to support optimal digestion and energy utilization.

7. Refuel Post-Workout:

- After a high-intensity workout on a high carb day, consume a post-workout meal or snack rich in carbohydrates and protein to replenish glycogen stores and promote muscle recovery.

8. Avoid Excessive Sugars:

- While high carb days allow for more carbohydrates, avoid excessive sugar consumption. Choose complex carbs over sugary treats to provide sustained energy without causing blood sugar spikes and crashes.

9. Customize to Your Goals:

- Tailor your high carb days to your specific objectives. If you're focusing on fat loss, high carb days should still be within your overall calorie goals, ensuring a caloric deficit for the week.

10. Be Mindful of Digestive Health:

- High carb days may include more fiber-rich foods. If you're not accustomed to a high-fiber diet, gradually increase fiber intake to avoid digestive discomfort.

High carb days are an opportunity to replenish glycogen stores, maximize energy levels, and support your workouts. By following these guidelines, you can make the most of these days within your carb cycling plan and move closer to your fitness and health goals.

5.2 Low Carb Days

Low carb days are an essential component of carb cycling, designed to promote fat loss and metabolic flexibility by reducing carbohydrate intake. Here's how to effectively implement low carb days:

1. Determine the Frequency:

- Decide how often you'll have low carb days in your carb cycling plan. The frequency can vary based on your goals, but it's typically around 1-3 times per week, depending on your activity level and objectives.

2. Choose the Right Carbohydrates:

- While you're reducing carbohydrate intake on low carb days, focus on consuming high-quality, non-starchy vegetables, leafy greens, and small portions of low-glycemic fruits like berries. These provide essential nutrients, fiber, and minimal impact on blood sugar.

3. Balance with Protein and Healthy Fats:

- On low carb days, increase your intake of protein and healthy fats to compensate for the reduction in carbohydrates. Protein supports muscle maintenance, and fats provide energy and satiety.

4. Monitor Carbohydrate Content:

- Pay attention to the carbohydrate content of foods. Avoid grains, bread, pasta, sugary snacks, and starchy vegetables on low carb days. Instead, choose lean protein sources like chicken, fish, tofu, and healthy fats like avocados, nuts, and olive oil.

5. Stay Hydrated:

- Maintain proper hydration on low carb days. Drinking enough water is essential for overall health and can help control hunger and cravings.

6. Manage Portions:

- Be mindful of portion sizes to avoid overeating. Since carbs are restricted, portion control is essential to stay within your calorie goals.

7. Time Your Low Carb Days:

- Plan low carb days on days when you have less intense or no workouts, as your energy requirements will be lower. These days can also be beneficial for promoting fat utilization.

8. Maintain Fiber Intake:

- Although you're reducing carb intake, aim to maintain adequate fiber intake by including non-starchy vegetables and leafy greens. Fiber supports digestive health and helps control hunger.

9. Monitor Blood Sugar Levels:

- If you have concerns about blood sugar levels or diabetes, consider monitoring your blood sugar response to low carb days and adjusting your carb intake accordingly.

10. Be Mindful of Your Body:

- Pay attention to how your body responds to low carb days. Some individuals may feel more fatigued, while others may experience improved mental clarity. Adjust your plan based on how you feel and your performance in workouts.

Low carb days are an opportunity to promote fat loss and enhance metabolic flexibility. By following these guidelines, you can effectively implement low carb days within your carb cycling plan while working toward your fitness and health goals.

5.3 Refeed Days

Refeed days are a crucial component of carb cycling, providing your body with a higher intake of carbohydrates to replenish glycogen stores and support overall well-being. Here's how to effectively implement refeed days:

1. Determine the Frequency:

- Decide how often you'll have refeed days in your carb cycling plan. The frequency can vary based on your goals and preferences but is often scheduled around every 1-2 weeks. Refeed days serve as a psychological and physiological break from low carb days and can help prevent metabolic adaptation.

2. Choose Quality Carbohydrate Sources:

- Prioritize high-quality, complex carbohydrates for refeed days. opt for whole grains like brown rice, quinoa, and oats, starchy vegetables like sweet potatoes, and fruits like bananas. These provide sustained energy and essential nutrients.

3. Time Your Refeed Days:

- Schedule refeed days strategically. They are often positioned on days when you have demanding workouts or when you're starting to feel the effects of low carb days, such as reduced energy or mental clarity.

4. Balance with Protein and Healthy Fats:

- On refeed days, ensure you consume adequate protein and healthy fats to maintain a balanced diet. Protein supports muscle maintenance and growth, while fats provide satiety and essential nutrients.

5. Monitor Portions:

- While you're increasing carbohydrate intake on refeed days, still be mindful of portion sizes to avoid overconsumption. Overeating can lead to excessive calorie intake, which may hinder your progress.

6. Stay Hydrated:

- Maintain proper hydration on refeed days. Drinking enough water is crucial for overall health and can support optimal digestion and energy utilization.

7. Avoid Excessive Sugars:

- While refeed days allow for more carbohydrates, avoid excessive sugar consumption. Choose complex carbohydrates over sugary treats to provide sustained energy without causing blood sugar spikes and crashes.

8. Enjoy Variety:

- Use refeed days as an opportunity to enjoy a wider variety of foods and flavors. Explore new recipes and incorporate foods you may have limited during low carb days.

9. Mindful Eating:

- Pay attention to your body's hunger and fullness cues on refeed days. Mindful eating can help you avoid overeating and maintain a healthy relationship with food.

10. Track Your Progress:

- Keep a food diary or use a mobile app to track your food intake on refeed days. This can help ensure you're meeting your nutritional and caloric goals.

Refeed days serve as a beneficial aspect of carb cycling, providing physical and psychological relief from low carb days while replenishing glycogen stores. By following these guidelines, you can effectively implement refeed days within your carb cycling plan and work toward your fitness and health goals.

5.4 Sample Carb Cycling Meal Plans

Creating sample carb cycling meal plans can be highly personalized, as they depend on individual preferences, dietary restrictions, and specific goals. However, I can provide you with three sample carb cycling meal plans for a better understanding of how to structure your meals on high carb, low carb, and refeed days. These meal plans are based on a 2,000-calorie daily intake but can be adjusted to your calorie and macronutrient needs.

Sample High Carb Day Meal Plan (2,000 Calories):

Breakfast:

- Scrambled eggs with spinach and tomatoes

- Whole-grain toast

- A small serving of mixed berries

Mid-Morning Snack:

- Greek yogurt with honey and a sprinkle of almonds

Lunch:

- Grilled chicken breast with quinoa

- Steamed broccoli and carrots

- Side salad with vinaigrette dressing

Afternoon Snack:

- A banana with almond butter

Dinner:

- Baked salmon with a side of brown rice

- Roasted asparagus and bell peppers

Sample Low Carb Day Meal Plan (2,000 Calories):

Breakfast:

- Omelette with mushrooms, spinach, and feta cheese

- Sliced avocado

Mid-Morning Snack:

- Cottage cheese with cherry tomatoes

Lunch:

- Turkey lettuce wraps with a side of sliced cucumber

Afternoon Snack:

- Celery sticks with hummus

Dinner:

- Baked cod with a side of steamed broccoli and cauliflower

- A small green salad with olive oil dressing

Sample Refeed Day Meal Plan (2,000 Calories):

Breakfast:

- Whole-grain pancakes topped with mixed berries and a dollop of Greek yogurt

Mid-Morning Snack:

- Trail mix with nuts, dried fruits, and a few dark chocolate chips

Lunch:

- Quinoa and black bean salad with mixed vegetables

- Grilled chicken breast with barbecue sauce

Afternoon Snack:

- Sliced apples with peanut butter

Dinner:

- Whole-grain pasta with tomato sauce, lean ground turkey, and a side of garlic bread

- Roasted Brussels sprouts

These sample meal plans illustrate how to structure your meals on high carb, low carb, and refeed days. Remember to adapt these plans to your specific goals, dietary preferences, and any dietary restrictions you may have. Additionally, consider consulting with a registered dietitian or nutritionist to create a personalized carb cycling plan that best suits your needs.

CHAPTER 6

Monitoring Your Progress

6.1 Tracking Your Macros

Monitoring your macronutrient intake is a critical aspect of tracking your progress in a carb cycling program. Here's how to effectively track your macros:

1. Calculate Your Macronutrient Targets:

- Determine the specific macronutrient ratios for your high carb, low carb, and refeed days based on your goals and caloric needs. Tools like nutrition calculators or guidance from a registered dietitian can help with this.

2. Use a Food Scale:

- Invest in a kitchen food scale to measure and weigh your food accurately. This ensures you're consuming the right portion sizes.

3. Read Food Labels:

- Pay attention to food labels to understand the macronutrient content of packaged foods. This is particularly useful for tracking carbohydrates, protein, and fat.

4. Use Nutrition Apps or Software:

- Utilize nutrition tracking apps or software, such as MyFitnessPal or Cronometer, to log your daily food intake. These tools can

provide a breakdown of your
macro and calorie intake.

5. Keep a Food Diary:

- If you prefer a manual approach,
  maintain a food diary where you
  record everything you eat and
  drink. Make note of portion
  sizes, cooking methods, and the
  macronutrient content of each
  item.

6. Be Consistent:

- Consistency in tracking is key.
  Record your food intake every
  day, whether it's a high carb, low
  carb, or refeed day. This helps
  ensure you're meeting your
  macronutrient goals consistently.

7. Adjust as Needed:

- Monitor your progress and be
  ready to adjust your

macronutrient targets if you're not seeing the desired results. Consult with a nutrition expert if you're unsure about the necessary changes.

6.2 Measuring Your Results

Measuring your results is essential to assess the effectiveness of your carb cycling plan and make necessary adjustments. Here's how to measure your progress:

1. Scale Weight:

- Regularly weigh yourself at the same time of day and under consistent conditions, such as in the morning after waking up and using the bathroom. Keep in mind that weight can fluctuate, so look for trends over time.

2. Body Measurements:

- Take measurements of your body, including your waist, hips, chest, arms, and legs. Track changes in these measurements to gauge progress in body composition.

3. Body Composition Analysis:

- Consider using methods like skinfold calipers, bioelectrical impedance scales, or DEXA scans to assess your body fat percentage and muscle mass. These provide a more accurate picture of changes in your body composition.

4. Performance Metrics:

- Monitor your athletic or fitness performance, such as the weights you lift, your running times, or your endurance during workouts. Improved performance can be an indicator of positive progress.

5. Energy Levels:

- Pay attention to your energy levels, mood, and overall well-being. Increased energy, better mood, and improved sleep quality can be signs of successful carb cycling.

6. Clothing Fit:

- Notice how your clothing fits. Looser-fitting clothes or the ability to wear smaller sizes can be a tangible sign of progress.

7. Photos:

- Take periodic photos to visually document changes in your physique. Comparing photos side by side can help you see changes that may not be immediately apparent in the mirror.

8. Consistency and Patience:

- Understand that results may not be immediate, and consistency is crucial. Give your carb cycling plan time to work and make adjustments as needed based on your progress.

Progress can vary from person to person, and what works for one individual may not work for another. It's essential to be patient, adapt your plan based on your results, and consult with a healthcare professional or registered dietitian if you have any concerns or questions about your progress.

6.3 Adjusting Your Plan as Needed

Adjusting your carb cycling plan as needed is a critical aspect of achieving your goals and maintaining a sustainable approach to nutrition and fitness. Here are some guidelines on when and how to make adjustments:

1. Monitor Your Progress:

- Regularly assess your progress through tracking your macros, measuring your results, and staying mindful of your energy levels, mood, and overall well-being. Look for trends over time, rather than focusing on daily fluctuations.

2. Be Patient:

- Understand that achieving significant results may take time. Allow your carb cycling plan to work for several weeks before making major changes.

3. Consider Your Goals:

- Revisit your initial goals and make sure they are still relevant and attainable. Your objectives may change over time, so your plan should align with your current aspirations.

4. Adjust Your Macronutrient Ratios:

- If you're not seeing the desired results, consider modifying your macronutrient ratios. For instance, on low carb days, you can decrease carbohydrate intake and increase fat and protein consumption.

5. Modify Meal Timing:

- Adjust the timing of your high carb, low carb, and refeed days based on your training schedule and energy needs. For instance, you may benefit from shifting high carb days to coincide with particularly challenging workouts.

6. Increase or Decrease Caloric Intake:

- If your weight loss or muscle gain has plateaued or you're experiencing excessive energy deficits or surpluses, adjust your overall caloric intake. On high carb days, you may need to increase calories slightly, while on low carb days, you can decrease them.

7. Seek Professional Guidance:

- If you're uncertain about how to adjust your carb cycling plan or if you're experiencing challenges, consider consulting with a registered dietitian, nutritionist, or fitness expert. They can provide tailored recommendations and guidance.

8. Experiment and Document Changes:

- Consider making one change at a time to your carb cycling plan. For example, you might modify your macronutrient ratios or meal timing and monitor the impact over a few weeks before making additional adjustments.

9. Listen to Your Body:

- Pay attention to how your body responds to changes in your plan. If you experience unusual fatigue, extreme hunger, or other concerning symptoms, this may be a sign that your plan needs further adjustment.

10. Be Flexible:

- Remember that no single approach works for everyone. Be open to adaptation and experimentation as you learn more about how your body responds to carb cycling and different nutritional strategies.

The key to successful carb cycling is finding a plan that suits your individual needs and is sustainable in the long term. Adjusting your plan as needed allows you to fine-tune your approach and continue making progress toward your health and fitness goals.

CHAPTER 7

Tips for Success

7.1 Staying Consistent

Consistency is crucial for the success of any dietary and fitness plan, including carb cycling. Here are some tips to help you stay consistent with your carb cycling program:

1. Plan Ahead:

- Plan your meals and workouts in advance. Knowing what to eat and when to exercise reduces the likelihood of making impulsive decisions that can disrupt your carb cycling plan.

2. Use a Food Diary:

- Maintain a food diary to track your daily intake and ensure you're following your macronutrient targets. There are many apps available that can make this process easier.

3. Meal Preparation:

- Prepare your meals in advance, especially for low carb days when you might be tempted to make less healthy choices due to time constraints.

4. Set Realistic Goals:

- Establish achievable, realistic, and specific goals. Unrealistic expectations can lead to frustration and a lack of motivation.

5. Accountability:

- Share your goals and progress with a friend, workout partner, or support group. Having someone to hold you accountable can be motivating and help you stay on track.

6. Be Mindful:

- Practice mindful eating by paying attention to your body's hunger and fullness cues. Avoid emotional or stress-related eating.

7. Monitor Your Progress:

- Regularly track your macros, take measurements, and assess your results to ensure you're moving in the right direction. Celebrate your successes along the way.

8. Adapt to Your Lifestyle:

- Make sure your carb cycling plan aligns with your daily routine and lifestyle. It should be sustainable and not feel like a burden.

9. Flexibility:

- Be adaptable and open to making necessary adjustments to your plan when needed. Life events, holidays, and unforeseen circumstances can affect your routine, so flexibility is key.

10. Stay Positive:

- Maintain a positive attitude. Understand that progress may not always be linear, and setbacks are a part of any journey. Learn from challenges and keep moving forward.

11. Learn from Mistakes:

- If you have a day where you deviate from your plan, don't dwell on it. Instead, learn from

the experience and use it as
motivation to stay on track in the
future.

12. Seek Support:

- Consider seeking guidance from
a registered dietitian or nutrition
expert who can provide tailored
advice and address your specific
needs and concerns.

13. Rest and Recovery:

- Remember that rest and recovery
are essential for your overall
well-being. Overexertion and
insufficient sleep can affect your
ability to stay consistent and
achieve your goals.

14. Enjoy the Journey:

- Embrace the process and enjoy
the journey. Focus on the
positive changes you're making

in your life and how they contribute to your overall well-being.

Staying consistent with carb cycling may require effort and discipline, but the rewards in terms of improved health, fitness, and well-being can be well worth it. By following these tips, you can maintain your commitment to your carb cycling plan and work towards your desired outcomes.

7.2 Dealing with Cravings

Managing cravings is a common challenge when following a carb cycling plan. Cravings can be triggered by various factors, including stress, emotional triggers, or a desire for comfort foods. Here are some strategies to help you deal with cravings effectively:

1. Identify the Cause:

- Recognize the root cause of your cravings. Are they linked to emotions, stress, or specific situations? Understanding why you have cravings can help you address them more effectively.

2. Stay Hydrated:

- Sometimes, thirst is mistaken for hunger. Drink a glass of water when you experience cravings to see if they subside.

3. Balanced Meals:

- Ensure your meals are balanced with adequate protein, healthy fats, and fiber-rich foods. Balanced meals can help control hunger and cravings.

4. Portion Control:

- If you're craving a particular food, consider allowing yourself a small, controlled portion to satisfy the craving without derailing your plan.

5. Substitute Healthier Options:

- Find healthier alternatives to satisfy cravings. For example, if you're craving something sweet, opt for fruit instead of sugary snacks.

6. Distract Yourself:

- Engage in an activity that can take your mind off cravings. Go for a walk, practice a hobby, or call a friend for a chat.

7. Practice Mindfulness:

- Mindful eating involves being fully present when you eat, savoring each bite, and paying attention to the tastes and textures. This can help reduce overeating and cravings.

8. Plan Ahead:

- If you know that certain times of the day trigger cravings, plan a healthy snack or meal for those moments to prevent succumbing to unhealthy options.

9. Keep Craving Foods Out of Reach:

- If you have specific trigger foods that you tend to overindulge in, keep them out of your immediate environment to reduce temptation.

10. Manage Stress:

- Practice stress-reduction techniques like meditation, deep breathing, or yoga to help

prevent emotional eating
triggered by stress.

11. Reward Yourself:

- Allow yourself an occasional
  treat as a reward for sticking to
  your carb cycling plan. This can
  help satisfy cravings while
  maintaining consistency.

12. Support System:

- Share your goals and challenges
  with a friend or family member
  who can provide support and
  encouragement during moments
  of temptation.

13. Be Kind to Yourself:

- Understand that occasional
  cravings and indulgences are a
  part of a balanced lifestyle. Don't
  be too hard on yourself for

giving in occasionally. Focus on
your overall progress.

14. Consider Nutrient Timing:

- Schedule high carb days or
  refeed days strategically to
  coincide with times when you
  typically experience strong
  cravings. This can help satisfy
  your desire for certain foods
  within the context of your plan.

Cravings are a normal part of the
human experience, and it's okay to
indulge occasionally in moderation.
The key is to find a balance that allows
you to meet your goals while still
enjoying the foods you love.

7.3 Exercise and Carb Cycling

Exercise plays a crucial role in the success of your carb cycling plan. It can help you achieve your fitness and health goals more effectively. Here's how to incorporate exercise into your carb cycling routine:

1. Align Workouts with Carb Cycling Days:

- Match your workout intensity with your carb cycling days. On high carb days, consider scheduling more demanding workouts, such as resistance training or high-intensity interval training (HIIT), to take advantage of the extra energy from carbohydrates. On low carb days, opt for lower-intensity exercises or rest days to accommodate reduced energy levels.

2. Pre-Workout Nutrition:

- On high carb days, consume a balanced meal or snack with a moderate amount of carbohydrates 1-2 hours before your workout. This provides fuel for your training session. Include some protein and healthy fats for sustained energy.

3. Post-Workout Nutrition:

- After a high-intensity workout on a high carb day, have a post-workout meal rich in carbohydrates and protein to replenish glycogen stores and support muscle recovery. This can help minimize muscle soreness and improve performance in subsequent workouts.

4. Resistance Training:

- Incorporate resistance training into your exercise routine. Building lean muscle can boost your metabolism and help you achieve your fitness and body composition goals.

5. Cardiovascular Exercise:

- Include cardiovascular exercises such as running, cycling, or swimming to improve cardiovascular health and burn calories. You can adjust the intensity and duration based on your goals and carb cycling phase.

6. Listen to Your Body:

- Pay attention to how your body responds to workouts on low carb days. If you find yourself feeling excessively fatigued, consider reducing the intensity or duration of your exercise or incorporating more rest days.

7. Adapt to Goals:

- Tailor your exercise routine to align with your goals. If you're primarily focused on fat loss, a combination of cardio and resistance training can be effective. If you're aiming for muscle gain, prioritize resistance training.

8. Maintain Consistency:

- Consistency in your exercise routine is key to long-term success. Stick to a regular schedule and incorporate workouts into your daily or weekly routine.

9. Cross-Training:

- Consider cross-training to prevent boredom and plateaus. Variety in your workouts can also help target different muscle groups and improve overall fitness.

10. Rest and Recovery:

- Ensure you incorporate rest days into your exercise plan to allow your body to recover and prevent overtraining. Rest is essential for muscle repair and overall well-being.

11. Hydration:

- Stay well-hydrated before, during, and after your workouts. Dehydration can negatively impact your performance and recovery.

12. Consult a Fitness Professional:

- If you're new to exercise or have specific fitness goals, consider working with a fitness professional, such as a personal trainer or fitness coach, who can create a customized workout plan.

The relationship between exercise and carb cycling should be flexible and adaptable to your specific goals and individual preferences. The key is to maintain a balance that supports your overall health and well-being while helping you achieve your desired outcomes.

7.4 Potential Pitfalls to Avoid

While carb cycling can be an effective strategy for achieving various health and fitness goals, there are potential pitfalls to be aware of and avoid. Here are some common pitfalls and how to steer clear of them:

1. Extreme Restriction:

- Pitfall: Going to extremes with very low-carb days can lead to nutrient deficiencies, reduced energy levels, and muscle loss.

- Solution: Ensure that even on low carb days, you're still consuming an adequate amount of carbohydrates to support your body's basic needs. Be mindful of extreme restrictions.

2. Neglecting Protein and Fats:

- Pitfall: Focusing solely on carbohydrates and neglecting protein and healthy fats can hinder muscle maintenance, metabolism, and overall health.

- Solution: Balance your macronutrient intake by incorporating lean protein sources and healthy fats into your diet on all carb cycling days.

3. Overindulging on Refeed Days:

- Pitfall: Treating refeed days as "cheat days" and overindulging in high-carb, high-calorie foods can counteract the benefits of carb cycling.

- Solution: While refeed days offer more flexibility, still make mindful choices and aim to satisfy cravings with healthier options that align with your goals.

4. Inadequate Hydration:

- Pitfall: Neglecting proper hydration can lead to reduced

energy, poor workout performance, and potential health issues.

- Solution: Ensure you stay well-hydrated by drinking water throughout the day, as proper hydration is crucial for all aspects of your health and fitness.

5. Ignoring Nutrient Quality:

- Pitfall: Focusing solely on macronutrients and ignoring the quality of the foods you consume can lead to nutrient deficiencies and health problems.

- Solution: Emphasize whole, nutrient-dense foods in your diet, including fruits, vegetables, lean proteins, and whole grains.

6. Overtraining:

- Pitfall: Pushing yourself to exercise excessively, especially on low carb days, can lead to burnout, injury, and diminished results.

- Solution: Balance your exercise routine, incorporate rest days, and adjust workout intensity based on your energy levels and carb cycling phase.

7. Neglecting Fiber Intake:

- Pitfall: Inadequate fiber intake can lead to digestive issues on low carb days.

- Solution: Incorporate non-starchy vegetables, leafy greens, and fiber-rich foods into your meals to support digestive health.

8. Relying Solely on Carb Cycling:

- Pitfall: Thinking that carb cycling alone is a magic solution can lead to disappointment. Other factors like overall calorie intake, sleep, and stress management also play important roles.

- Solution: Approach carb cycling as one element of a comprehensive health and fitness plan. Consider how it fits into your overall lifestyle.

9. Unrealistic Expectations:

- Pitfall: Having unrealistic expectations about the speed of results can lead to frustration and disappointment.

- Solution: Set realistic and achievable goals, and understand that meaningful changes often take time.

10. Skipping Professional Guidance:

- Pitfall: Attempting carb cycling without consulting a healthcare professional or registered dietitian, especially if you have specific health concerns, can lead to issues.

- Solution: Seek guidance from a qualified expert to ensure that your carb cycling plan aligns with your needs and goals.

Avoiding these pitfalls and staying informed about the potential challenges of carb cycling can help you implement this nutritional strategy more effectively and safely. Remember that everyone's body is unique, and what works best for you may require some experimentation and adaptation.

7.5 Next Steps on Your Carb Cycling Journey

Now that you've learned about carb cycling, it's time to take the next steps on your journey. Here's a guide on what to do next:

1. Set Clear Goals:

- Define your specific health and fitness goals. Whether it's weight loss, muscle gain, improved athletic performance, or enhanced overall well-being, having clear objectives will guide your carb cycling plan.

2. Consult a Professional:

- Consider consulting with a registered dietitian, nutritionist, or fitness expert. They can provide personalized guidance and help you create a carb

cycling plan tailored to your
needs.

3. Customize Your Plan:

- Use the knowledge you've
  gained to create a carb cycling
  plan that suits your goals,
  lifestyle, and preferences. Adjust
  macronutrient ratios, meal
  timing, and workout routines
  accordingly.

4. Start Slow:

- If you're new to carb cycling,
  ease into it by gradually
  incorporating high carb, low
  carb, and refeed days into your
  routine. This allows your body to
  adapt and prevents
  overwhelming changes.

5. Track Your Progress:

- Continue to monitor your progress through tracking macros, measuring results, and staying mindful of your energy levels. Regularly reassess your goals and make adjustments as needed.

6. Experiment and Learn:

- Carb cycling is not one-size-fits-all. Experiment with different approaches to find what works best for you. Be open to learning from your experiences and making necessary adjustments.

7. Stay Consistent:

- Consistency is key to success. Stick to your carb cycling plan and exercise routine, and prioritize healthy choices on all days, not just on specific carb cycling days.

8. Be Patient:

- Understand that meaningful results may take time. Be patient with yourself, and don't be discouraged by occasional setbacks.

9. Seek Support:

- Share your journey with friends or join a support group to stay motivated and accountable. It can be helpful to have a community that shares similar goals.

10. Continue Your Education:

- Stay informed about the latest research and nutritional information related to carb cycling. As science evolves, so does our understanding of optimal dietary strategies.

11. Adapt and Evolve:

- Your goals and needs may change over time. Be prepared to adapt and evolve your carb cycling plan to align with your current circumstances and aspirations.

12. Enjoy the Process:

- Embrace your carb cycling journey as a path to better health and well-being. Enjoy the process of learning more about your body and how it responds to different nutritional strategies.

Carb cycling is a dynamic and flexible approach to nutrition that can help you achieve your health and fitness goals while promoting balance and sustainability. Keep an open mind, be adaptable, and use the knowledge you've acquired to embark on a successful carb cycling journey.

www.ingramcontent.com/pod-product-compliance
Lightning Source LLC
Chambersburg PA
CBHW070818280726
48660CB00016B/2126